CBD

OR

CANNABIDIOL

CBD & Cannabis Medicine;
Essential Guide to Cannabinoids
and Medical Marijuana

Aaron Hammond

By Aaron Hammond
Version 2.2
Published by HMPL Publishing at KDP
Get to know your publisher and his work at:
http://happyhealthygreen.life

A personal note from the writer

I have been involved in the cannabis scene and the medical benefits of marijuana for a long time. That's why writing this book was more than just a pleasure. Cannabis use has been on the rise and with the increasing amount of positive results from research about cannabinoids, I jumped to the opportunity of sharing this information about CBD and other cannabinoids with you.

I will teach you the basics of what those cannabinoids do to our bodies and brain, how that can be beneficial to us, and a future medicine with tremendous value. I have been a recreational user of cannabis for more than 10 years now; I have problems with my back and in the last year I experienced the amazing pain relieving effects of CBD first hand.

To provide you with the best information, I wrote this book as unbiased, objective and informative as possible. It was hard to not 'sell' it as a miracle medicine with so many positive results and medical benefits popping up in the news.

I hope that in the future CBD and medical marijuana will change our approach to issues in the medical world. Legalization is key and will make it possible for more and more people to benefit from medical marijuana.

With kind regards,

Aaron Hammond

or blame be held against the publisher for any reparation, damage, or monetary loss due to the information herein, either directly or indirectly.

Respective authors own all copyrights not held by the publisher. The information herein is offered for informational purposes solely, and is universal as so. The presentation of the information is without contract or any type of guarantee assurance. The trademarks that are used are without any consent, and the publication of the trademark is without permission or backing by the trademark owner. All trademarks and brands within this book are for clarifying purposes only and are owned by the owners themselves, not affiliated with this document.

Table of Contents

Bonus

Welcome to HMPL Publishing! Let's start right away with an exclusive bonus made available only for our inner circle.

Get your free eBook **'The best DIY THC & CBD recipes to prepare at home'** here: http://eepurl.com/cxpVZf

Subscribing to our newsletter will get you the latest THC and CBD recipes, articles and some of our upcoming eBooks for absolutely free. To make that even better we'll update you with the most recent information about marijuana, medical breakthroughs, and the various applications of cannabis.

You can visit also
http://happyhealthygreen.life

Or connect with us on Facebook;
https://www.facebook.com/happyhealthygreen.life

CBD – A Short Introduction

CBD stands for cannabidiol. It is a substance found in the cannabis and hemp plants. Until recently CBD was not in the spotlight like its counterpart, also found in the cannabis plant – THC. However, recently, with more research coming to light about CBD and its role along with THC, there is renewed attention coming and turning the tides on the persistent stigma that has surrounded cannabis use.

All this while marijuana, a Schedule I drug, has been looked upon only from a recreational standpoint, and been deemed illegal for it. It wasn't until recently, that a number of states in the United States have started to legalize marijuana for both medical and recreational use.

The turn of the tide is not just observable in the US. The UK has also started to mobilize, and plans are underway to review the legalization of cannabis for medical use. Canada is already fully on board. There is also positive news from countries in Europe. And in the Netherlands and Spain, it has been legal to use for quite some time now.

When we broach the legal framework that surrounds marijuana, we begin to understand that there are larger issues which need to be understood and categorized to come up with a fair and beneficial perspective on the issue. In this quest, we need to figure out the nature of CBD and THC. From there we need to understand how each of the two substances affects the body and the brain. How they work together, and how they work in isolation. We will look at this as we travel through this book.

* * *

Important Medical Disclaimer

(Please read: CBD and/or THC together or individually can have side effects when consumed along with other compounds, medications, and substances. Please seek professional advice!)

Many people choose to self-medicate, and to a certain extent, that's fine. However, in many cases, one substance can and will react with another substance. Sometimes that reaction could be positive, but that's hardly the experience. In most cases, contraindications between substances exist and will have adverse effects on the patient.

If you are a patient of a serious condition such as epilepsy, cancer, COPD, or some other serious disease or condition where CBD and THC could have great medical potential, you should discuss it with your medical practitioner to see how CBD interacts with your current medication.

Cannabidiol Contraindications

When a patient consumes pharmaceutical drugs, it has to be metabolized by the body, and that is done by the liver. More than 50% of a compound metabolized by the liver is done so by the enzyme cytochrome -p450. When a patient consumes CBD, that CBD inhibits the enzyme cytochrome-p450 and that blocks the ability of the body to effectively metabolize the other medication.

Here is a list of most common drugs that are affected in this way. These drugs are known to be metabolized by cytochrome p-450:

- Steroids
- HMG CoA reductase inhibitors
- Calcium channel blockers
- Antihistamines
- Prokinetics
- HIV antivirals
- Immune modulators
- Benzodiazepines
- Antiarrhythmics
- Antibiotics
- Anaesthetics
- Antipsychotics
- Antidepressants
- Anti-epileptics
- Beta blockers
- PPIs
- NSAIDs
- Angiotensin II blockers
- Oral hypoglycemic agents
- Sulfonylureas

Please understand that this list is not complete but we named what is known right now. In addition to that, individuals can react differently and some may or may not have reactions like the others. It is for this reason that you should seek advice from a medical professional when considering cannabidiol or if you feel that you have reduced cytochrome P-450 functionality.

A major issue that proponents and potential CBD users is the negative stigma towards CBD or cannabis use that can stain professional medical advice.

You will find methods of extraction in this book. Use them as a guide but continue to seek advice from medical professionals if you have serious health concerns. The methods used yield specific concentrations; varying even a little can have an effect on that and thereby on the dosages that you consume. It cannot be stressed enough that you need to find an unbiased professional to have the best results of the information that you extract from this book.

The entire point of this book is to provide easy-to-understand information. It is not a scientific journal nor a rigorously peer-reviewed publication. It is, however, a very thoroughly researched collection of data and methods that seek to explain the subject matter to the widest possible audience. For those of you who are interested in scientific sources, you will find a list of papers and studies which you can refer to, all of which will back up the information given.

Lab tested CBD products can be expensive, ranging in prices above $700 for 3600 mg of pure CBD. This is beyond the reach of many of the folks who would be best served by it. This is a significant setback in obtaining and using CBD.

Another obstacle is the legal environment that you are under. It may be illegal in your jurisdiction to purchase or consume cannabis or its related products. Whatever the problem may be, there is something in this book for you to be able to overcome it.

The main goal of this book was to process all the scientific information out there and focus on the importance of CBD, while keeping it simple for everyone. After all, cannabis is easily grown as you can find in our grow guide for beginners, if you know how, and the extraction of the useful compounds is not that much more difficult. So why should all the data and methods be covered in secrecy by the companies that make them?

There is no reason for it and this book is written to break that.

This book will remain as an introduction to the many options that exist. Further in-depth books are planned and will be written to follow the information laid out here.

* * *

Understanding CBD

The human body contains a central and peripheral nervous system that has, among other things, an endocannabinoid system (ECS) throughout its network of nerves. The endocannabinoid system is made up of cannabinoid receptors found along the entire length of your nervous system, from the brain to the rest of your body.

As far as scientists can tell; there are over 113 compounds in the cannabis plant that can be extracted. A compound found in cannabis is categorized as a cannabinoid when it is able to attach to the cannabinoid receptors in the human ECS. Two popular cannabinoids from the many compounds found in the cannabis plant are cannabidiol, CBD; and, tetrahydrocannabinol, THC; while the lesser known cannabinoids include cannabichromene (CBC), cannabinol (CBN), and cannabigerol (CBG).

There are two species of cannabis plants that are the primary source of the cannabinoids discussed here – Cannabis sativa and Cannabis indica. What we normally refer to as hemp (Cannabis Ruderalis) is part of the sativa family but has a noticeable difference in the ratio of THC and CBD compared to cannabis.

Cannabis has been grown over the years for its THC and CBD but hemp pretty much remained the same as the plant materials are needed for industrial production. So there has never been much change in the containment of cannabinoids and the levels of THC and CBD are notably lower.

THC is a psychoactive compound whereas CBD is a non-psychoactive compound found in cannabis. CBD was first discovered in 1940 but the chemical structure and stereochemistry were specified more than 20 years later in 1964.

Studies conducted in the last 30 years have shown how CBD and THC inhibit potent medicinal benefits. We have come to learn a lot about what CBD does in terms of positive effects whereas the negative effects remain mostly insignificant.

* * *

Cannabinoids and how they work?

Phytocannabinoids are cannabinoids that are derived from plant sources, as opposed to endocannabinoids that are synthesized within the body. The two most popular phytocannabinoids are tetrahydrocannabinol (THC) and cannabidiol (CBD). Both can be extracted from the cannabis or hemp. From the cannabis plant, scientists have been able to find over 113 compounds including CBD and THC. But cannabis plants are not the only source of cannabinoids. Cacao is an example of another plant that contains certain cannabinoids. It should be noted that neither of those cannabinoids found in cacao are THC or CBD.

The main characteristic of cannabinoids is that they have an affinity to attach to and influence certain cells in the human body. Cannabinoids will attach to cells with a cannabinoid receptor in them. When the cannabinoid attaches to a certain cell in the brain, that cell is then instructed to do something. For instance, when THC is introduced into the bloodstream, it attaches itself to cannabinoid receptors that primarily involved with the release of the dopamine neurotransmitter.

The human central and peripheral nervous system beginning in the brain and extending throughout the body contains cannabinoid receptors. These receptors are able to bind with some of the many cannabinoids produced by the cannabis plant, or with endocannabinoids from our own body.

There are two receptors in particular which play major roles in the effect cannabinoids have on the body. The two primary receptors are simply named Cannabinoid Receptor Type 1 and Cannabinoid Receptor Type 2. Also known as CB1 and CB2, respectively. Human beings are not the only ones that possess CB1 and 2 receptors and the endocannabinoid system. Other mammals, birds, fish, and reptiles also possess the ECS.

Cannabinoid Receptors Type 1

The cannabinoid receptor type 1 is primarily located in the central and peripheral nervous system. These receptors are activated by the endocannabinoid neurotransmitters known as anandamide and 2-arachidonoglycerol and plant cannabinoids such as the compound THC. These receptors can also be found in the lungs, liver and kidneys. The main function is the mediation of certain neurotransmitters known as acetylcholine, noradrenaline, dopamine, 5-HT, GABA, glutamate, D-aspartate, and cholecystokinin.

In the liver, the receptor is responsible for increasing novo lipogenesis, or better said, turning your carbohydrates into fatty acids. Presynaptic Cb1 receptors in your liver are responsible for guarding your blood pressure by activation in certain situations.

CB1 Lowers Anxiety and Stress

In tests using mice that did not have CB1 receptors, researchers noticed that they were visibly more anxious and upon deeper physical inspection found that they had a larger amygdala. Each brain has an amygdala located in the temporal lobe. The amygdala is primarily responsible for regulating a number of powerful emotions including fear and motivation. That points to the conclusion that CB1 Receptors are important in balancing and controlling anxiety, more so during periods of high stress.

Additionally, the location of the high concentration of CB1 receptors in the area, specifically in and around the amygdala and the neighbouring hippocampus have a bearing on emotional responses and how emotions are triggered and prolonged. It also has a significant bearing on memory and mood stability. Thus it has been widely theorized and in some cases practiced, that exciting these CB1 receptors have a positive effect in the amygdala region and the hippocampus thereby providing a remedy to mood disorders, emotional imbalances and issues we know as bipolarity, ADHD, and similar psychiatric issues.

The CB1 receptors in the brain tend to impact systems that rely on the GABA/Glutamate balance. GABA and Glutamate are neurotransmitters that work in opposition to each other and when in balance all is normal. GABA is a calming neurotransmitter while glutamate is an excitatory neurotransmitter. More of one and less of the other doesn't necessarily result in better or worse states. But rather their levels when regulated properly by the body serve important functions. In the event of inflammation or when your immune system needs to kick in, you will find that there is increased glutamate activity. When everything is working well, then GABA increases to counter the effects of glutamate with the objective of maintaining homeostasis. CB1 receptors are found on GABA and glutamate neuron terminals seem to be able to control their release and thereby control the GABA/glutamate balance. In almost the same way, CB1 has an effect on dopamine transmitters in the release of dopamine. It also has an effect on serotonin. Dopamine, if you recall is the feel-good neurotransmitter and floods your brain with pleasure. While serotonin regulates mood, anxiety, and happiness. Low serotonin levels result in depression and possible anxiety. Which is why CB1 agonists like endocannabinoids (cannabinoids produced by the body) can excite them as can phytocannabinoids like delta-9-tetrahydrocannabinol (THC).

Drugs That Block Cannabinoid Receptors

The cannabinoid receptor is open to both cannabinoids produced within the body and ones that are taken from outside sources. It doesn't really differentiate between the two. Imagine the receptor (CB1 or CB2) as the keyhole in a lock, and when the key, in this case, the cannabinoid, is able to enter and turn, it unlocks the cell. One way for the key to not affect the lock would be to block the keyhole. When that happens, the key is unable to enter the lock and have any effect. This is one way of reducing the efficacy of the cell, and of the receptor. In trials, the effect of blocking the receptor can be observed in the increase (up to three times more) in anxiety symptoms when a cannabinoid blocker is introduced. In some cases, there is even a serious onset of depression. Once the regimen of cannabinoid blockers was stopped, trial subjects returned to normal within 24 hours. The drug that blocked the CB1 receptor had an effect of making people more negative and even reduced their pleasure when experiencing things that would normally give them pleasure. The CB1 blocker drug also activated the HPA axis.

The HPA, hypothalamic - pituitary - adrenal, axis is a set of control and feedback between the three glands in the endocrine system and results in, among other things, controlling the digestive system, reaction to stress, sexuality, and the control of energy usage.

CB1 and Post Traumatic Stress Disorder (PTSD)

Stress in human beings, or in any animal for that matter is a series of chemical interactions. Strong evidence points to the fact that the cannabinoid system plays a major role in keeping stress at appropriate levels and either aiding in the adaptation of stress or in the buffering of it.

Cannabinoids are not just external substances that influence our neurophysiology. There are naturally occurring cannabinoids within the ECS. One of them is anandamide. Anandamide, known as N-arachidonoylethanolamine or AEA, is a ligand that attaches to CB1. When the subject is faced with psychological stress, anandamide levels in the limbic regions that are involved with emotion and cognition are observed to decrease. The decrease is even more aggressive in the amygdala.

In a recent study, researchers found that levels of anandamide and 2-Arachidonoylglycerol (2-AG) to be significantly lower in those suffering from

PTSD. This was event the case when compared to those who had suffered trauma but not developed PTSD in its wake.

The reduced AEA can also result in the release of cortisol during events of psychological stress. Typically, the reduction in anandamide lasts for 24 hours from the point of the stressful event.

Cannabinoid Receptors Type 2

We know that CB1 receptors are found primarily in the brain, although they are found in other areas of lower concentration. CB2, on the other hand, are found in lower concentrations in the brain but in higher concentrations in one specific system in the human body-- the immune system. In the brain, they are predominantly located in the microglia. From the spleen to the thymus gland and including the tonsils there is increased levels of CB2 receptors that when activated are predominantly responsible for inhibition of cytokine release. CB2 receptors are also found on the family of immune cells including T-cells, B-cells, macrophages, and monocytes. You can also find them on mast cells.

Mast cells, or mastocytes, are cells that are part of the immune system that, when triggered, are involved in the production and release of histamine and heparin. CB2 receptors located on the mast cell control its performance and thereby have an impact on their function thereby having a direct impact on how often and how much histamine and heparin are released into the body.

In the intestinal tract, CB2 is also found where they function to limit intestinal inflammation. This makes CB agonist potential sources of relief for bowel diseases such as Crohn's and colitis.

CB2 receptor agonists (the molecule that fits in the receptor) can cause a reduction in the intracellular levels of cyclic adenosine monophosphate (cAMP). When there is a reduction in cAMP, it results in the reduction of CREB, a binding transcription factor that causes changes in the genes which regulate the immune system. This then results in the successful suppression of the immune system.

For patients with Alzheimer's, neural functioning is disrupted by the build-up of plaques, made of beta-amyloid proteins. The role CB2s play here are important as they can activate the macrophages, cells that 'eat' other cells, that destroy the plaque that is disrupting the normal neuron firing process. It has been shown that activation of these receptors has strong ability to counter Alzheimer's.

One of the most astounding revelations from studies conducted in the various medical fields spanning different disciplines is that almost every ailment induced in the human body shows a change in endocannabinoid levels. Whether it is gastrointestinal, psychiatric, cardiovascular, endocrine, neurological or dermatological, they all have potential cures in CB2 activation and control.

It has even been found that CB2 receptors can be activated to reduce cocaine addiction.

* * *

What does CBD do exactly?

Cannabidiol has no psychotropic effects like its counterpart THC. In fact, CBD is able to neutralize the effects of THC to a certain extent and when taken together CBD acts as a counterbalance to THC in the 'high' that the consumer experiences.

CBD attaches to both the CB1 and the CB2 receptors in the body and serves as discussed above, as a counter towards THC. This makes CBD a formidable ally in countering the effects of the other cannabinoids. In realistic terms, this means that the consumption of CBD gives us the benefits of cannabinoids without the psychotropic effects of THC and one of the other hundred compounds of the cannabis plant.

There is research that has shown that CBD also has an effect on serotonin levels, adenosine levels as well as glycine and vanilloid receptors (these are responsible for body temperature and feel the effect of heat-related pain). In the event of fire-related injuries, CBD can be used as a relief for pain caused by the burn.

CBD also has a potent antidepressant function. It has been found that CBD is involved in the stimulation of 5-HT1A serotonin receptor that is known to produce the antidepressant effect.

This receptor also has bearing on appetite, pain perception, nausea, anxiety, and addiction mechanisms.

Finally, it has also been found that CBD can reduce the proliferation of cancerous cells and bone resorption by inhibiting GPR55 signalling. GPR55 is dominant in the brain and is associated with controlling blood pressure, modulating bone density, and preventing the proliferation of cancerous cells.

We will discuss more about that when we get to the health benefits of CBD and how you can use it as a medicine.

* * *

Medical Use and Application

CBD has the following medical properties we currently know:

- ➤ Antiemetic (reduces nausea and vomiting)
- ➤ Anticonvulsant (suppresses seizure activity)
- ➤ Antipsychotic (combats psychosis disorders)
- ➤ Anti-inflammatory (combats inflammatory disorders)
- ➤ Antioxidant (combats neurodegenerative disorders
- ➤ Anxiolytic/Antidepressant (combats anxiety and depression disorders)

CBD as an Anticonvulsant

Studies over the last decade that show the effectiveness of CBD as an anticonvulsant. CBD actively reduces the severity of seizures in animal trials. There have also been case-studies on the effects of CBD on children with drug-resistant types of epilepsy suggesting potential treatment using CBD.

CBD as Anti-inflammatory

Numerous studies report that CBD has neuroprotective properties in cell cultures proving that it has positive repercussions on neurodegenerative diseases such as Parkinson's, MS, and Alzheimer's. It has also shown promise in repairing brain damage caused by alcohol abuse.

Recent clinical trials have shown that substances containing CBD have been successful in treating spasticity associated with MS.

For those with Parkinson's disease sleep quality is a major issue and CBD has shown to be able to increase and improve sleep quality. CBD has been able to vastly improve complex sleep behaviours associated with rapid eye movement (REM), promptly reducing the symptoms of the disorder and helping to improve sleep quality.

CBD as an Anxiolytic/Antidepressant

It is no secret that cannabis has the potential to induce acute psychotic episodes at high doses under certain circumstances, and several studies have shown that marijuana use increases the risk for chronic psychosis in individuals with associated genetic risk factors. Several studies and clinical trials have suggested that THC mediated those effects, and it has been suggested that CBD counteracts as an anti-psychotic and is capable of mitigating the psychotic effects of the THC. There have been a few small-scale clinical trials over the past time where patients with psychotic symptoms were treated with CBD, including case reports of patients with schizophrenia. There has been a small case study in patients with Parkinson's disease with psychosis, which reported positive results after treatment with CBD; and one small randomized clinical trial reporting clinical improvement for patients with schizophrenia who took CBD over a certain amount of time. Large randomized clinical trials would be needed to be fully able to evaluate the therapeutic potential of CBD for patients with schizophrenia, bipolar disorder and other forms of psychosis.

CBD has also been able to show, in recent studies, that it is capable of reducing anxiety and stress, by reducing both behavioural and physiological (e.g., heart rate) symptoms of stress and anxiety in animal models. In addition, small-scale human laboratory and clinical trials have provided evidence that CBD has shown to be beneficial and efficient. The reports of those trials prove that CBD is able to reduce stress and anxiety in patients with social anxiety.

In a laboratory protocol designed to model post-traumatic stress disorders, CBD has improved "consolidation of extinction learning", in other words, patients were able to forget traumatic memories. The anxiety-reducing effects of CBD appear to be triggered by altering the serotonin receptor 1 signalling, although more research is needed to fully understand this mechanism.

* * *

Can Cannabinoids Treat Cancer?

The International Cannabinoid Research Society has been responsible for the organizing efforts and bringing together the research in the thrust to push cannabinoid research in the forefront of cancer research. Original research in this area began in the late 60s and early 70s. Between then and now, volumes of research papers resulted from the process of researching cannabinoids as an effective solution to cancer, or cancer treatment.

If you want more information there are numerous publications put out by credible sources, including The Welcome Witness, all make for interesting reading, detailing the history and politics cannabis in medicine. Nature, another scientific journal, was another publication that published quite a few reviews on cannabis.

The one point that needs to be made is that, while there are numerous journals, thousands of blogs, and many publications on the possibility of using cannabis to treat and cure cancer, this is, by far, not solid proof. Any attempt to frame it as such would be categorically misleading. To understand the role of cannabinoids and cancer, you need to take a hard look at the evidence.

Lab Research

The biggest factor that is unknown to casual readers has to do with the way lab tests and research are done. It is a fact that a very high number of tests, virtually all, investigations into the viability of cannabinoids to treat cancer was conducted using lab-made cells or done with animal models. These results were then extrapolated to human conditions. When it comes to medicine, it is very dangerous to consider something works conclusively when it is only extrapolated results. What's more, almost all the relevant research has been performed in various labs without any real-life testing. The human system is significantly more complex than whatever you can cook up in labs or even compared to living specimens like mice. But it does not stop there. Whatever research that has been done. Even the ones that were done in labs could not find conclusive evidence. What they did find is summarized as follows:

- ➢ *Triggering apoptosis* - or otherwise known as cell death
- ➢ *Halting the automatic division of cells*
- ➢ *Prevention of new blood cell growth*
- ➢ *Reducing cancerous cells from spreading*
- ➢ *Speeding up autophagy* - the process of cell destruction

Research seems to suggest, and this is not all

fully proven yet, that cannabinoids locking on to CB1, CB2, and other receptors are at the centre of all these effects.

Among all the various combinations, the optimal results in lab tests and animal trials have been found to come from the use of combining THC and CBD. Remember, CBD counterbalances some of THC's effects especially its negative effects (psycho activity). There are positive outcomes, researchers have found that the use of cannabinoids from synthetics sources, such as the molecule JWH-133. JWH-113 is a compound discovered by John W Huffman that selectively attaches itself to CB2 receptors and is responsible for the prevention of inflammation in Alzheimer's as well as the prevention of cognitive markers.

But be warned, there are also drawbacks, side effects, and undesirable consequences to taking on a cannabis medicine in the fight against cancer.

For instance, one of the drawbacks of THC is that in very high doses it can damage cells of the vessels that carry blood in the process. Although these high doses can potentially kill cancer, when taken to reduce or reverse cancer cells, it is possible to end up damaging healthy blood vessels. This is also seen in the fact that THC stops the growth of blood vessels to the cancerous cells as well, starving these cells of the nutrients they need.

Surprisingly, it has also been reported that under certain circumstances, cannabinoids can actually encourage cancer cell growth. Studies have discovered how activation of the CB2 receptors by cannabinoids may enhance the immune defences against cancer. It is also possible that the cancer cells become immune to cannabinoids and begin advancing again.

However, it seems that a better alternative to battle cancer is to combine THC with other conventional cancer therapies know today and allow them to work in union. That has proven to be a lot more effective. It could be a better option to use cannabinoids as a supplement with different chemotherapy regimens. Experiments in the lab seem to support that if cannabinoids were combined with drugs like temozolomide as well as gemcitabine, the outcome could be very positive.

Whenever research regarding cannabis and cannabinoids hits the news, there is a lot of interest on social media. But this often turns out that the hype doesn't actually reflect the work done. For example, a recent study from researchers at the University of East Anglia was done using cancer cells grown in the lab or transplanted into mice, to try and understand why different levels of purified THC seem to have different effects on cancer cells – something that has been noticed from previous experiments on cannabinoids and cancer cells. The researchers found that THC works through two different receptor molecules coming together – CB2 and GPR55 – and that high doses slow cancer cells growth while low doses don't. So they think that designing drugs that make sure the receptors come together in the right way to kill cancer cells could be a good way to harness the potential power of cannabinoids to treat cancer in a much more effective and targeted way.

But while this is definitely an interesting scientific paper and helps to shed light on the "nuts and bolts" that underpin how certain cancer cells may respond to cannabinoids, and could point to ways to make cannabinoid drugs more effective in the future, this certainly doesn't tell us that cannabis can be used to effectively treat cancer in patients at the moment.

Clinical Research

Lab studies show a much less conclusive result. One trial that has been testing cannabinoids on cancer patients was done in Spain. The trial was headed by Dr. Manuel Guzman and a team of scientists. A total of nine patients diagnosed with terminal stages of glioblastoma multiforme were prescribed doses of THC in its highest purity. This was injected directly into the brain.

Eight of those patients responded, while the ninth didn't. However, every single one of them passed away. It showed nothing different from what was expected in terms of fatality rate and time. That study showed us that THC can be safe and seemingly without any complications, but you must keep in mind that it was not a conducted with control groups.

While encouraging, the results cannot be taken to mean anything conclusive. The trial seems to point to the fact that cannabinoid research towards cancer is definitely worth pursuing. But it is far from conclusive yet the rumours and stories seem to suggest that cannabis is a cure. It does no good to spread or listen to stories that are not verified about possible cures. Unless there is a strong basis in science throughout their trials whatever is said is based more on hype and half-truths. Information like this should not be relied upon and should not be propagated.

Unanswered Questions

The greatest doubt that is cast over the debate is on the things that we yet do not know. There is some evidence that points positively toward cannabinoids, but there are more questions than there are answers.

One of the main issues is that we are not certain which sort of cannabinoid to use - natural, synthetic, endocannabinoid or phytocannabinoid.

We are not sure which is more effective, or what dosage levels we should be looking at. What confuses everything even more, is that different forms of cancer tend to react differently to different cannabinoids. This results in one simple analysis - that there is no universal conclusion to be made for cancer in general. Each one is unique and requires specific solutions.

It's true that most research and publicity has surrounded the use of THC. But new research and new findings also show that other kinds of cannabinoids may have better results in different strains of cancer. THC is no longer the only game in town with it comes to having hopes for a cure for cancer.

Aside from this, there is also the psychoactive nature of THC. The other cannabinoids don't seem to have the same psychoactive result as THC does and in many cases that are preferable. Between the stigma of it and the illegality of it, THC causes more of a hurdle than it does provide solutions.

There is also a problem in getting the compounds into the actual tumour sites. The compound is not entirely water-soluble and is not able to travel long distances when passing human tissue. Delivery, if it is to be effective needs to be directly transported to the site of the tumour, which means it could require an invasive procedure - each time a dosage is administered.

The Guzman trial we talked about earlier in Spain conducted the trials by injecting the cannabinoids directly into the patient's brain. The procedure was highly invasive and ultimately proved to be unsuccessful. It is also unknown at this stage if cannabinoids would help or hinder regular chemotherapy by boosting or counteracting the primary attack against cancer cells.

Can Cannabis Prevent or Cause Cancer?

Instead of hoping that it could cure cancer, is there a possibility that cannabis could maybe prevent it? If we ask that question, we also have to ask if there is the potential that it could cause other kinds of cancer. The point is we do not yet know any of this.

In mice, the studies have shown that the larger doses of THC had the potential of decreasing the levels of risk against having certain kinds of cancer develop. This, coupled with the fact that some cannabinoids (especially ones developed internally) have the ability to suppress tumour growth, gives us hope that phytocannabinoids could do the same.

On the other hand, we have longstanding evidence from usage since the 80s where drugs made from cannabinoids were successfully used to combat some of the symptoms patients experienced from chemotherapy. This included severe cases of nausea and vomiting. Drugs such as dronabinol and nabilone were widely used back then to make the course of chemotherapy less difficult. That is still the case in Holland today where marijuana for medicine is legalized for pain relief and adverse symptoms. The problem has been with dosing, and that has not yet been accurately established.

Sativex

Sativex is a mouth spray. Currently in the United Kingdom, trials have been commissioned to test this product. This is a concentrated extract of pharmaceutical quality, containing both tetrahydrocannabinol (THC) and cannabidiol (CBD). This mouth spray could assist in controlling pain caused by cancer.

It is also suggested that cannabinoids could be used to overcome appetite loss and the subsequent depression. Tests are underway but the results have not yet showed proof of the theory. There are published results from trials of using Sativex on glioblastoma multiforme, combined with temozolomide, showing increased survivability rates in patients. The same results were obtained from another test as well. While promising, extensive trials that are more sophisticated are required to determine its efficacy and if cannabis can proceed to the next stage.

Just Because Cannabis Is Natural Doesn't Make a Cure

Nature holds many compounds that can be used within the human body to bring it into balance or throw it out of balance. Some have great medical potential while others can diminish vitality and even cause fatality.

Taking something natural for one issue can yield side effects in other areas. Some side effects are small, while other can be complex. But it does not mean just because it is natural, that it is healthy or beneficial. Cyanide, can also occur naturally and we know that that is not healthy by any means.

In fact, certain fungi can yield medical benefits. This was the inspiration and starting points for the development of penicillin and other antibiotics. It does not mean we can harvest fungus and consume them to counter a bacterial infection.

Another example is aspirin. It comes from the bark of the willow. If taken in its natural form it could cause complications like severe irritation of the bowels. But the inspiration caused a pharmaceutical company to develop acetylsalicylic acid. It works the same but does not affect the stomach.

Cancer Drug Development

By taking inspiration from nature, even cancer drug developers can find solutions to complex problems. One of the ways is to take something that occurs naturally then purifying it and targeting it for a specific purpose. For instance, take the leaves of the yew plant. That resulted after some ingenious tinkering to become the drug known as Taxol. In the same way there is Vinblastine that was inspired by Rosy Periwinkles, and Camptothecin that came from the Xi Shu tree. Even the May Apple resulted in Etoposide. What's really interesting is that a common spice found in Indian curries -- turmeric -- has the ability to treat bowel cancer when it's curcumin is extracted in its pure form.

The key to remember is that just because something in high doses can have an effect does not mean that its source plant is able to yield the same results. Just because high doses of THC can have a positive effect, it doesn't mean the cannabis plant is the cure for cancer.

"Have you seen this video? This guy says cannabis cures cancer!"

It's easy to get carried away by the hype across the internet on how there is a cure for cancer in cannabinoids and marijuana. There are tons of anecdotal accounts of cures and such, but none of them are able to stand up to medical grade research. So it would be wise to read carefully what one has to write.

The bottom line is that whatever they say and claim, you must realize that this is not scientific evidence.

Before you place any hope in a claim for effective treatment of cancer, you should make sure that it is clinically proven. Otherwise, you are just setting yourself up for additional pain and headaches down the line.

We all agree that it is in our global interest to find a cure for cancer. To get to that point researchers need to conduct rigorous medical research and trials. Organizations that base their work on research need outcomes that are solid and based on facts and evidence. It is vital that we stick to the facts and results based on solid research since what is at stake is nothing less than life.

"What's the harm? There's nothing to lose."

The harm is this. If someone believes the misinformation on cannabinoid treatment for cancer, and gives up on regular treatment in favour of something unproven, then their death and suffering during cannabis treatment is the direct result of the misinformation. The conventional treatment may not have saved them, but it may have lengthened their life. It is important to say that cannabis treatment can be effective in a way that conventional treatment fails to do, but it is a complete gamble as every patient is unique and cannabis is not (yet) a cure for cancer.

It is widely accepted that natural cannabinoids are mostly safe for human consumption, the problem is in combining them with other medications. Contraindications are a problem.

Some stories also can be scary. Like the one about the Dutch lung cancer patient who used cannabis that he purchased on the street and slipped in a coma within hours due to the fact that someone had laced his cannabis with harmful chemicals.

Preparations made at home, or ones found in black markets can come with high risks because the method of extraction is unsure and could be contaminated with pesticides and chemicals that are cheap and dangerous. Because most preparation methods use solvents in the process, they are usually the cause for toxicity depending on the type and grade of solvent used. It is even possible that if the cannabis plant originally contained harmful pesticides, that may be further condensed in the process and increase its toxicity.

More importantly, you must know that there are many trying to just make a buck. On the streets and on the internet. For that buck they will promise you the world and deliver products that are useless at best, or toxic at worse. There are some good sources, but the majority do not fall into this category. For this reason, be very careful who you listen to and from where you buy products.

The best place to get advice is from your trusted medical professional and find out if medical marijuana is an option. If you live in a legal state or country, a patients' license to use and grow marijuana is your best bet. This is a great way of getting access to good cannabis that could possibly make a difference.

* * *

How to Apply CBD?

The previous sections have shown what CBD is and how CBD works. That gives you the ability to see the advantages, disadvantages, potential and risks. As far as medical potential, CBD has definitely shown tremendous promise.

With that behind us we are able to move to the next step and explain the different ways we can use CBD.

The first step is to understand how to find CBD. The most common way you can find it is in the form of CBD hemp oil. This can be further narrowed down into edibles, oils, tinctures, and topicals. However, you can get highly concentrated CBD oil as well. You can find most of these products in the US and Europe. You can get these from a number of online retailers, pharmacies, apothecaries, and dispensaries. Some places require a medical prescription, others do not. It depends on the jurisdiction that you and the seller are in.

The one thing that surprises most people is when they find out that the use of cannabis-based products is personalized. Each person has their own dosage depending on a number of factors based on the person's metabolism and the reason they are taking the CBD in the first place.

To achieve the maximum benefit from cannabis, make sure to choose your cannabis products that include both CBD and THC because these two compounds enhance each other providing the best medical effects and therapeutic effects. The key factor in determining the correct ratio and dosage of CBD-rich medicine is your sensitivity to THC. There are many people who enjoy the high that THC in cannabis provides and can consume reasonable doses of any cannabis product without getting a feeling that they're too high or uncomfortable. But there is a possibility that you might find the effects of THC unpleasant. As we explained in earlier chapters CBD is able to counteract the intoxicating effects of THC. The right balance between THC and CBD levels is your first step to getting effective treatment with cannabis products.

So you need to find the right balance between CBD and THC levels for you. That balance varies from one person to the next. It is possible to take a mixture where you have no negative side effects from THC if you can find the right balance. Each person is different; each person's needs are different and each person will react differently to different ratios. That is the main point of all of this.

If you suffer from spasms, anxiety, depression, or pediatric seizure disorders, there are many patients who initially find they get the best treatment from a moderate dose of a CBD-dominant product (a CBD/THC ratio of more than 10:1). But treating your condition or disease with a product that has a low level of THC, while not intoxicating, is not always the best option for treatment. Sometimes a combination of CBD and THC will most likely have a greater medical effect for a wider range of conditions than CBD or THC alone.

For cancer, neurological disease, and many other ailments, conditions and diseases, there are patients that may benefit from a balanced ratio of CBD and THC. There has been extensive clinical research that has shown how a 1:1 CBD/THC ratio is very effective for neuropathic pain. Optimizing your medical use of cannabis should be approached carefully and can be a step by step process where you try to get the best possible balance of THC/CBD ratio in your medicine that fits the condition you're treating. This gives you the option to start with small doses of a non-intoxicating CBD-rich cannabis product, observe the results, and gradually try to increase the amount of THC. Simply put, the goal is to self-administer consistent, measurable doses of CBD medicine that includes as much THC as a person is comfortable dealing with.

* * *

Dosing

CBD oil brands tend to create a lot of confusion for consumers because they all have different standards of consumption and dosing. Many of these brands recommend way too much as a "serving" and others recommend too little. I would personally recommend to start using 25mg of CBD twice a day.

It is also recommended that you try increasing your dosage every 3-4 weeks by 25mg until symptom relief. If you find symptom relief within these small doses you don't have to increase. You will need to decrease the amount of CBD if there is any worsening of your symptoms. This will tell you if the CBD is causing it. Concentrations of CBD oils, extracts and concentrates may vary between preparations for medical use, ranging from 1 mg per dose to hundreds of milligrams. This makes it easy for you to get the dosages you need in a form that you find easy to use.

➢ To increase appetite in cancer patients: 2.5 milligrams of THC by mouth with or without 1 mg of CBD for six weeks

➢ To treat chronic pain: 2.5-20 mg CBD orally for an average of 25 days

> To treat epilepsy: 200-300 mg of CBD taken orally daily for up to 4.5 months

> To treat movement problems associated with Huntington's disease: 10 mg CBD per kilogram of body weight by mouth daily for six weeks

> To treat sleep disorders: 40-160 mg CBD by mouth.

> To treat Multiple Sclerosis symptoms: Cannabis plant extracts containing 2.5-120 milligrams of a THC-CBD combination oral daily for 2-15 weeks. A mouth spray might contain 2.7 milligrams of THC and 2.5 milligrams of CBD at doses of 2.5-120 milligram for up to eight weeks. Patients typically use eight sprays within any three hours, with a maximum of 48 sprays in any 24-hour period.

> To treat schizophrenia: 40-1,280 mg CBD oral daily for up to four weeks

> To treat glaucoma: a single CBD dose of 20-40 mg under the tongue. Doses greater than 40 mg may actually increase eye pressure.

There is no established lethal CBD dose but I urge you to read product disclaimers very carefully to ensure that you are taking the right amount of CBD and talk to your medical practitioner about any questions or concerns.

How is CBD Hemp Oil Used to Create CBD Products?

Farms that grow cannabis for the production of concentrated CBD products have harvests of their high-CBD/low-THC strains where they will put their buds and plant materials through a specialized solvent-free extraction process to yield a hemp-oil that has a high concentration of cannabidiol. This pure cannabis extract then has to be tested for safety, quality, and cannabinoid content before they get processed in CBD products or hit the shelves directly as a concentrate. When it comes to CBD products in the US where cannabis yet has to be legalized in 21 states and medical use is allowed in 29 states; import can be your only option; depending on where you live. CBD is legal but you will have to extract it from industrial-grade hemp if you want to make it yourself and that process is not legal depending on who you're asking at the DEA. This makes CBD usually very expensive for states where importing it is the only option you have, so be sure to support legalization if you think that this needs to be changed.

* * *

Making Your Own CBD Oil

This is an urgent message for anyone considering the use of this method to extract their own CBD. Since you are working with alcohol as a solvent it is of the utmost importance that you are aware of your surroundings. Be aware of open fires, stoves, smoking and other situations that could catch fire!

Before you start: Measuring CBD containments

The safest way of measuring how many milligrams of CBD your extract contains is to have it lab tested. But that is not always an available option. So here is a simple trick if you're in a situation where you need to measure it yourself.

Understand that this method of measurement will not be the most accurate but it will help to indicate purity and dosage starting out with the plant material.

I would recommend using only buds that are medical grade cannabis if not for recreational purposes and buy them from certified dispensaries or farms.

Now provided that you have the choice between several different strains with the tested THC/

CBD levels, you want to pick the strains that contain high CBD levels and low THC levels for CBD oil extraction. For people who are completely new to this; let me explain that THC levels are independently different compared to CBD levels; 1-5% THC is considered to be a very low level of THC while 1-5% CBD is fairly high for a strain, so at the very high end of THC levels you should be looking at 20-30% THC per gram, whereas the strains with a high CBD level are around 15-20% CBD. These amounts of compounds in cannabis are a key point in breeding new strains of medical marijuana to grow buds with higher THC/CBD levels.

What you should be looking at as a good CBD oil extract is a good CBD strain that has been tested with high levels of CBD ranging from 5-20% while THC remains at 5% and preferably much lower. If you are growing marijuana yourself THC/CBD levels should be provided with the seeds of your strain, if you're getting them from a professional cannabis seed company. They offer a great variety of high CBD/low THC level strains.

You have the choice to pick the seeds that fit your need of medical marijuana. If you prefer a different balance of compounds, for example; you want a high THC/very low CBD oil for daily use with the uplifting or relaxing effects of THC the same rules of measurements are applied.

It all comes down to this: 1% of a single gram is 10 milligrams; so if you have a strain that contains 15% THC and 2% CBD we're looking at 150 milligrams of THC and 20 milligrams of CBD. This is the way to measure the buds you are using. If they are lab-tested, THC/CBD levels will be provided. If this is not the situation and you didn't grow it yourself or there is no way of ever testing it, you can't say anything about it.

You can speculate THC and CBD levels by the effect of using this cannabis. It's a general fact that high THC and very low to almost no CBD and CBN containing strains tend to give an uplifting, energizing, positive and, possibly, an anxious effect. Whereas unknown strains or cannabis purchased illegally with higher CBD and CBN levels (at the very, very rare maximum of 2% CBD per gram) usually gets you stoned. These strains will work at relaxing, sedating, or give you a couch-lock and work great against stress and anxiety.

It is almost completely impossible to ever encounter a pure CBD strain as recreational drugs illegally on the streets as the effects are strictly medical and won't get you high. These 5-15% CBD/5% and lower-THC strains will not make you feel high or stoned as CBD doesn't inhibit a psychoactive effect and it counters the psychoactive effect provided by the small amount of THC completely. The best way to get those strains is at your local dispensary or to grow them yourself.

Personally, I cannot recommend ever buying marijuana illegally because it usually hasn't been tested; this cannabis bears the risks of containing pesticides or powders such as calcium, milk powder, and other materials to improve the weight. There is a chance that glass-like glossy chemicals such as hairspray or simply glass powder have been used to make it appear like a densely THC covered bud.

There is a risk that your illegally purchased and untested cannabis could be contaminated with PCP or other chemical drugs to improve effects and could be potentially very dangerous! This has in no way to do with the plant itself but it is one of the dark sides of the drug business and a very urgent reason for legalization! Remind yourself that this part of the business is still illegal and usually doesn't have any concern for the user as there is money to be made.

Measuring the Contents of Cannabis Oil

Here is where it gets a little harder to get exact measuring on your own. If there is a possibility to get your oil lab-tested I urge you to do so as this method is not always very accurate. The larger the quantity of oil and used cannabis the easier it gets to measure the level of THC and CBD given that you have the right information. Because you will need to apply the same formula to calculate CBD and the amounts are easier weighted when they are larger.

So, for example, if you take a pound or 453 grams of lab-tested cannabis buds with 9.5% THC and 15.9% CBD you would technically have 43.035 grams of THC (95 mg of THC in a gram so 95 x 453: 1000 = 43.035 grams of THC in pound of buds). The same principle applies to calculating the amount of CBD where you take the 159 mg of CBD in a gram, multiply that by the amount of cannabis. So take 453 grams and divide the outcome through 1000 you should be looking at 72.027 grams of CBD in a pound of buds tested at 9.5% THC and 15.9% CBD. Now that we know this; you're looking a potential 100% pure return in oil that should be 114.052 grams.

This would be extraction done to perfection and nearly impossible to achieve without the proper experience and knowledge.

As we will be using cheesecloth to strain the plant material and raw bud to makes this oil you will have plant residue left in your oil which will bring the concentration down, but I have seen, tested, and used some very good homemade cannabis oils made by this method that got lab-tested at a level of 70-95% of purity.

We know what to look for now when you're making your own cannabis oil and want to measure the amounts of THC and CBD in your cannabis oil. But you want it to be exact. For example, you have tested your product so you're looking at 85% pure with 50% CBD and 35% THC in 100 grams of cannabis oil.

That means that you have about 15 grams of plant residue in your oil but the oil itself is very potent and of very high quality. If you know your math and if you're able to use the metric system this is will be very easy to calculate given that you are provided with the right information concerning the cannabis that you're using.

In one of my books I went in-depth into the world of cannabis extracts and concentrates as this is one of my passions and field of expertise.

* * *

How to make CBD oil?

This is an easy grain alcohol cannabis oil extraction method.

This process will yield you about 2 to 4 grams of extremely potent, medicinal-grade CBD or THC oil that is suitable for ingestion. After you have a few practice runs, the entire process for small-batch edible oil production should take you about an hour, including around thirty minutes of cooking time. Grain alcohol is the solvent that is least likely to leave you impurities or residue in the final product.

Supplies Needed:

> ➢ One ounce of dried, ground-up bud material or two to three ounces of ground, dried trim/shake

> ➢ One gallon of solvent (Grain alcohol or other high-proof alcohol; never use rubbing alcohol)

> ➢ Medium-sized mixing bowl (Glass is best, or ceramic)

> ➢ Strainer (A cheesecloth/stainless steel kitchen sieve combo, or muslin bags, grain-steeping bags or even clean stockings/nylons)

➢ Catchment container

➢ Double boiler or aubain Marie

➢ Kitchen utensils (Large wooden spoon, silicone spatula, plastic syringe for dosage and dispensing of oil, funnel)

Procedure:

1. Get organized – Prepare your space, arrange your necessary equipment, find a level work area and make sure that it is clean and set up before starting

2. Place the ground-up cannabis material into the mixing bowl, making sure to leave some space for the solvent. Find a larger bowl before proceeding further, if necessary.

3. Completely cover the plant material with the alcohol, adding about an extra inch of solvent above the top level of plant matter.

4. Using the wooden spoon, agitate the cannabis material within the solvent for about three minutes. This enables the resin glands to dissolve into the solvent. Make sure that the plant matter is thoroughly saturated and has had a chance to expel its resin content.

5. Place straining bag or sieve into the catchment container. Pour the dark green liquid from the mixing bowl into the bag or sieve; allow the liquid to be filtered completely and pour into the container. Gently massage the bag in order to squeeze out as much liquid as possible.

    Note: At this point, you have the possibility to repeat the previous four steps in order to extract as much resin as possible into the solvent. This second wash should remove most of the remaining resin.

6. Pour the strained liquid into the double boiler or in the cooking pots (au-bain Marie; placing a smaller cooking pot in a bigger one, allowing to put water in the bottom pot to prevent the top pot from overheating or cooking to quickly). Fill the bottom of the double boiler or the bottom pot with an appropriate amount of water. If your alcohol-resin solution does not all fit in the top of the double boiler or cooking pot, you can keep refilling the pot as you boil down the CBD oil, eventually processing all of the rinse liquid.

7. Place the double boiler on high heat until

the liquid begins to bubble, which is actually the alcohol evaporating. When it reaches the bubbling stage, turn off the burner – the residual heat contained in the water bath will continue heating the mixture, allowing the alcohol to evaporate.

8. If the mixture stops bubbling, it may be necessary to turn the heat back on, once or twice more. The evaporation step usually takes between fifteen and twenty-five minutes to complete.

   Note: The mixture should continue bubbling throughout the evaporation process. As the alcohol level decreases, so will the amount of bubbles. It helps to occasionally mix the solution with the silicon spatula, scraping the sides of the pan as you mix.

9. Do not let the mixture get too hot, as this will damage the cannabinoids and compromise potency and flavour. When the mixture is still runny but has stopped bubbling, turn the heat back on 'low', encouraging the mixture to begin bubbling again, then turn off the heat. Continue stirring, which will allow even more alcohol to evaporate away.

10. The oil is done when it has reached a thick, tar-like consistency and no longer bubbles. Since it continues to thicken as it cools, it is important to transfer the oil into storage or dosage containers at this point.

11. Slowly draw the CBD oil into the plastic syringes. As you reach the bottom of the pan, this will become more difficult, which is normal. Transfer any remaining amounts into small, air-tight containers. Aside from squeezing out small doses from the syringe, a toothpick can also be used to portion off dosages.

Note: If a topical application is preferred, simply combine the CBD oil with olive or coconut oil while it is still warm. This also decreases the potency, stretching out the dosages for cash-strapped or less experienced users.

Topical and Edible CBD Recipes

The possibilities with CBD oil are almost endless but we'd like to provide you with two very common recipes in which you can your cannabidiol extract. We'd like to show you a glimpse of those possible by showing how CBD oil is used in a DIY topical and the classic homemade CBD edible.

CBD-oil Topical: (Hand) balm

Enthusiasts swear by their use of CBD balm to treat all manner of ailments, including conditions such as rheumatoid arthritis, lupus, dermatitis, and psoriasis. When the (hand) balm is properly prepared, topical Cannabis balm can have analgesic, relaxing, anti-inflammatory, decongestant, and regenerative benefits, and such preparations of balm have been present in the human pharmacopeia for thousands of years.

Ingredients:
- ✦ -½ Ounce of cannabis with high CBD levels
- ✦ -½ cup of Shea butter, coconut oil, or beeswax (a combination of the three works best and is highly recommended)

Instructions:

1. Place the oils in a glass or ceramic mixing bowl. If you are using a combination, use a wooden spoon and mix them well.

2. Put a large pot on the stove and fill it halfway (or less) with water.

3. When the water is hot (but not boiling) put the mixing bowl in the pot. Be certain that no water gets inside the bowl.

4. When the oils have liquefied and are well blended, add your cannabis.

5. Continue to gently simmer, stirring every few minutes, for about 45 minutes. The longer it simmers the more potent your salve will be.

6. Strain the salve through cheesecloth into another glass container. Squeeze the cloth to get out every drop you can from the cannabis.

7. Allow the salve mixture to cool completely before using.

8. Once cooled, you can use a spoon or spatula to move your salve to a different container if you like.

9. Stored in a cool, dark place, your balm will keep for about 2 months.

Note: Adding some beeswax to your oil will help to make your (hand) balm firmer and more stable. Using only beeswax will leave you with a very hard substance which can be used as lip balm but be sure if you don't want that to add at least one other type of oil to the mix.

You can also add almond oil or grapeseed oil for a smooth, non-greasy type of balm. *

If you would like to have a sweet-smelling balm, add about a dozen or so drops of the essential oil of your choice. Mix them in with the other oils you have chosen.

CBD-oil Infused Edible

If you love cooking and getting creative in the kitchen this might be your thing. In this method to extract CBD oil from cannabis plant materials we noted that you can infuse this oil in either butter or coconut and olive oil. CBD-infused coconut and olive oil or butter is the defining ingredient to make your CBD-infused edible and a simple trick to see the possibilities of CBD-infused edibles is the given fact that in every recipe where you need to use butter or oil to bake or cook; you can use your CBD-infused oil or butter to prepare this recipe and make yourself some original homemade edibles.

Ingredients:

> 2 ½ Cup of flour, plus more for rolling

> 1 Cup sugar

> 1 Cup CBD-infused butter or coconut oil

> 1 egg

> 1 teaspoon baking powder

> 1 teaspoon vanilla

> 1 teaspoon salt

Optional: Powdered sugar and milk, for frosting

For less potent cookies, switch out any portion of the CBD infused butter and replace with standard butter as desired.

Instructions

1. Beat your CBD-infused butter or coconut oil, sugar, eggs and vanilla in a large bowl with a mixer on medium speed until thoroughly combined.
2. In a separate bowl, mix dry ingredients.
3. Add dry ingredients to your CBD-infused butter mixture a little at a time, stirring until all ingredients are incorporated.
4. Cover dough and refrigerate the mixture for the minimum of an hour or longer.
5. Remove dough from refrigerator and preheat oven to 180°C /375°F.
6. Roll dough on a generously floured surface to approximately ⅓ inch thick. Cut cookies by using a mug or cup upside down to press out some perfect circles and transfer to ungreased baking sheets.
7. Bake for 10-12 minutes or until lightly golden in colour.
8. Remove from oven, transfer to cooling rack and let cool completely before frosting.

To frost: Combine powdered sugar with milk and stir until desired consistency is reached, then add food colouring as desired.

Yield: Approximately 18 cookies.

Bonus

Welcome to HMPL Publishing! Let's start right away with an exclusive bonus made available only for our inner circle.

Get your free eBook **'The best DIY THC & CBD recipes to prepare at home'** here:
http://eepurl.com/cxpVZf

Subscribing to our newsletter will get you the latest THC and CBD recipes, articles and some of our upcoming eBooks for absolutely free. To make that even better we'll update you with the most recent information about marijuana, medical breakthroughs, and the various applications of cannabis.

You can visit also
http://happyhealthygreen.life

Or connect with us on Facebook;
https://www.facebook.com/happyhealthygreen.life

List of backing research papers

This is a list of all the titles of the researches used for this book. You may look them up by searching the full title of the research on Google as most of them are publicly available.

- Borgelt et al. The pharmacologic and clinical effects of medical cannabis.

  Pharmacotherapy 2013.

- Usar- Poli et al. Distinct Effects of Δ9-Tetrahydrocannabinol and Cannabidiol on Neural Activation During Emotional Processing.

  Arch Gen Psychiatry 2009.

- Jones et al. Cannabidiol exerts anti-convulsant effects in animal models of temporal lobe and partial seizures.

  Seizure. 2012.

- Consroe P and Wolkin A. Cannabidiol--antiepileptic drug comparisons and interactions in experimentally induced seizures in rats.

  J Pharmacol Exp Ther. 1977 - Apr;2011

◒ Gloss and Vickrey B. Cannabinoids for epilepsy.

Cochrane Database 2014.

◒ Iuvone et al.Neuroprotective effect of cannabidiol, a non-psychoactive component from Cannabis sativa, on beta-amyloid-induced toxicity in PC12 cells.

J Neurochem. 2004

◒ Hampson et al. Cannabidiol and (-)Delta9-tetrahydrocannabinol are neuroprotective antioxidants.

Proc Natl AcadSci U S A 1998.

◒ Russo EB. Cannabinoids in the management of difficult to treat pain.

Therapeutics and Clinical Risk Management 2008.

◒ Iskedjian et al. Meta-analysis of cannabis based treatments for neuropathic and multiple sclerosis-related pain.

Curr Med Res Opin. 23(1):17-24.(2007).

◒ Portenoy et al. Nabiximols for opioid-treated cancer patients with poorly-controlled chronic pain: a randomized, placebo-controlled, graded-dose trial.

J Pain. 2012 May;13.

- McAllister et al. The Antitumor Activity of Plant-Derived Non-Psychoactive Cannabinoids.

  J Neuroimmune Pharmacol. 2015.

- Wilkinson et al. Impact of Cannabis Use on the Development of Psychotic Disorders.

  Curr Addict Rep. 2014.

- Iseger and Bossong. A systematic review of the antipsychotic properties of cannabidiol in humans 2015.

- Guimaraes et al. Antianxiety effect of cannabidiol in the elevated plus-maze.

  Psychopharmacology 1990.

- Bergamaschi et al. Cannabidiol reduces the anxiety induced by simulated public speaking in treatment-naive social phobia patients.

  Neuropsychopharmacology 2011.

CPSIA information can be obtained
at www.ICGtesting.com
Printed in the USA
BVHW01s0929090218
507491BV00002B/161/P